HEALING WITH HORSES

Therapeutic Benefits, Equine-Assisted Therapy, And Emotional Healing Techniques For Personal Growth And Wellness

DR. MELISSA STOTLER

Copyright © 2023 by Dr. Melissa Stotler

Disclaimer:

The data in this book, is solely meant to be informative and instructional.

This book is not intended to replace expert medical advice, diagnosis, or care. No medical, health, or other professional services are offered by the author, publisher, or any affiliated parties

Individual outcomes may differ in the practice of these therapies, which entail a variety of approaches and methodologies.

A one-on-one session with a trained or certified healthcare professional is still preferable. It is best to consult a trained healthcare provider before making any decisions regarding your health.

The author of this book is not affiliated with any specific website, product, or organization related to any of these therapies.

All reasonable measures have been taken by the author and publisher to guarantee the authenticity and dependability of the material contained in this book.

Contents

ABOUT THE BOOK

Healing With Horses is a transformative guide that delves into the profound benefits of equine-assisted therapy, offering an unparalleled understanding of how horses can support healing and personal growth. This book begins by exploring the fundamentals of equine-assisted therapy, from its various forms and the meticulous process of selecting and training therapy horses to the pivotal roles played by therapists and horse handlers. With insights drawn from success stories and research findings, readers are introduced to the powerful impact this therapy can have on individuals seeking emotional and physical healing.

Preparation is crucial for making the most of therapy sessions, and this book provides detailed guidance on how to prepare for your first encounter with equine therapy. It covers essential aspects such as finding a qualified therapist, understanding what to expect during initial visits, and preparing both the horse and yourself for a successful therapy experience. Emphasis is placed on safety guidelines and mental preparation to ensure a smooth transition into this therapeutic journey.

Building a solid relationship with a horse is key to effective therapy, and this guide offers practical techniques for fostering trust and understanding between humans and horses. By focusing on horse behavior, body language, and basic handling skills, readers will learn how to create a positive interaction environment and develop a meaningful bond through engaging activities.

The book explores various equine-assisted therapy techniques, including groundwork, mounted activities, sensory and balance exercises, and therapeutic games. It highlights how these techniques can be tailored to meet individual needs, addressing both emotional and psychological issues such as anxiety, depression, and trauma recovery. By leveraging the unique capabilities of horses, individuals can build self-esteem, improve social skills, and track emotional progress.

The physical benefits of equine-assisted therapy are also thoroughly examined. From enhancing motor skills and physical strength to managing pain and supporting rehabilitation, this guide provides detailed information on how therapy contributes to overall physical health and endurance. Common challenges and solutions are discussed, offering practical advice on overcoming fear, managing behavioral issues, and adapting techniques for special needs.

Integrating equine therapy into daily life is another focus, with guidance on creating a routine, combining therapy with other treatments, and setting long-term goals. Readers will find valuable information on involving family and support systems to maintain and amplify the benefits of treatment beyond the sessions.

Lastly, the book addresses common concerns and provides detailed FAQs, covering topics such as the suitability of equine therapy, associated costs, and risk management. This comprehensive approach ensures that readers are well-informed and prepared to embark on a healing journey with horses.

CHAPTER ONE

UNDERSTANDING EQUINE-ASSISTED THERAPY

What is Equine-Assisted Therapy?

Equine-assisted therapy (EAT) is a therapeutic approach that involves interactions between a person and a horse to address physical, emotional, and psychological challenges. The therapy leverages the natural behaviors and instincts of horses to promote healing and growth in individuals. Through various structured activities and exercises, EAT aims to improve emotional well-being, physical coordination, and social skills.

During sessions, clients work with horses in a safe and controlled environment, engaging in activities such as grooming, leading, and riding. These interactions can help clients develop trust, build confidence, and learn new coping strategies. EAT is often used to support people with a range of issues, including anxiety, depression, PTSD, and developmental disorders.

Types Of Equine-Assisted Therapies

Equine-assisted therapy encompasses several types, each with its unique focus and methods. Here are the primary types:

Equine-Assisted Psychotherapy (EAP): This type involves a licensed mental health professional and a horse. Sessions are designed to help clients work through emotional and psychological issues by addressing their interactions with the horse. EAP can assist with trauma, anxiety, and relationship issues.

Equine-Assisted Learning (EAL): EAL focuses on personal development and life skills rather than addressing mental health issues. It often involves team-building exercises and problem-solving activities that help individuals develop communication skills, leadership qualities, and self-awareness.

Therapeutic Riding: This form of EAT uses horseback riding to improve physical and cognitive abilities. Therapeutic riding is particularly beneficial for individuals with physical disabilities, as it helps improve balance, coordination, and muscle strength.

Hippo-Therapy: Also known as Hippotherapy, this type uses the movement of the horse to provide physical therapy. It is conducted by licensed physical, occupational, or speech therapists who incorporate the horse's movements into their therapeutic goals.

How Therapy Horses Are Selected And Trained

Selecting and training therapy horses is a critical part of ensuring the success of equine-assisted therapy. Horses chosen for therapy roles must possess specific traits and undergo rigorous training:

Selection Criteria: Therapy horses are typically selected based on their temperament, behavior, and health. Ideal therapy horses are calm, patient, and responsive. They must be comfortable around people and able to handle various stimuli and environments without becoming stressed or reactive.

Training Process: Once selected, therapy horses undergo specialized training to prepare them for therapeutic sessions. This training includes desensitization to various equipment, exposure to different environments, and socialization with people. Horses are trained to respond to commands and maintain a calm demeanor during sessions.

Ongoing Evaluation: Therapy horses are continually evaluated to ensure they remain suitable for their roles.

Regular health check-ups, behavioral assessments, and training updates are essential to maintain their effectiveness in therapy.

The Role Of The Therapist And Horse Handler

In Equine-Assisted Therapy, both the therapist and the horse handler play crucial roles in facilitating effective sessions:

The Therapist: The therapist is typically a licensed mental health professional or a specialist trained in EAT.

They guide the therapeutic process, set goals, and help clients work through their issues using the interactions with the horse. The therapist also ensures that sessions are conducted safely and ethically.

The Horse Handler: The horse handler is responsible for the day-to-day care and management of the therapy horses.

They ensure that the horses are well-groomed, healthy, and properly prepared for sessions. The handler also assists in managing the horses during therapy, ensuring they remain calm and responsive.

Collaboration: Effective communication and collaboration between the therapist and the horse handler are essential.

They work together to design and implement therapeutic activities that meet the client's needs while ensuring the safety and well-being of both the horses and the clients.

Success Stories And Research Findings

Numerous success stories and research findings underscore the benefits of Equine-Assisted Therapy. These stories highlight the transformative impact EAT can have on individuals' lives:

Success Stories: Many clients report significant improvements in their emotional and physical well-being following EAT sessions.

 For example, individuals with PTSD have found relief through the calming presence of horses, while children with autism have developed better social skills and communication abilities.

Research Findings: Studies have demonstrated the effectiveness of EAT in various therapeutic contexts. Research shows that EAT can reduce symptoms of anxiety and depression, improve motor skills and balance, and enhance overall quality of life.

For instance, a study published in the Journal of Autism and Developmental Disorders found that therapeutic riding improved social interactions and motor coordination in children with autism.

These success stories and research findings provide compelling evidence of the value of Equine-Assisted Therapy, illustrating its potential to foster healing and personal growth.

CHAPTER TWO

PREPARING FOR YOUR FIRST SESSION

Embarking on your first equine therapy session can be both exciting and overwhelming. Here's how to make the process smoother:

Finding A Qualified Therapist

Finding the right therapist is crucial for a successful therapy experience. Start by researching practitioners in your area who specialize in equine-assisted therapy.

Look for certifications from reputable organizations such as the Professional Association of Therapeutic Horsemanship International (PATH Intl.) or the Equine Assisted Growth and Learning Association (EAGALA).

Read reviews from other clients to gauge their experiences. Don't hesitate to ask potential therapists about their qualifications, experience, and approach to therapy.

What To Expect During Your First Visit

During your initial visit, the therapist will likely conduct a thorough assessment of both you and your horse. They will discuss your goals, expectations, and any specific concerns you might have.

Expect to spend some time getting to know the facility, meeting the horses, and understanding the therapy process.

The session may start with groundwork or simple exercises to gauge the horse's and your comfort levels.

The therapist will guide you through each step, ensuring that both you and your horse are at ease.

How To Prepare Your Horse For Therapy

Preparing your horse for therapy involves ensuring they are calm, healthy, and comfortable. Begin by acclimating your horse to the therapy environment.

Spend time in the therapy area to help your horse become familiar with the surroundings. Make sure your horse is up-to-date on vaccinations and has a recent health check. Groom your horse thoroughly before the session, and ensure they are properly tacked up if necessary.

Bringing along familiar items, like their favorite brush or blanket, can help ease any anxiety they might feel.

Safety Guidelines For Therapy Sessions

Safety is paramount during therapy sessions. Always wear appropriate attire, including a helmet and gloves, to protect yourself.

Ensure that your horse is wearing well-fitting tack and is in good health. Follow all instructions from your therapist and maintain a calm demeanor to avoid startling the horse. Be aware of your surroundings, and keep the therapy area clean and free of hazards.

If you have any concerns about the safety protocols, discuss them with your therapist before the session begins.

Preparing Yourself Mentally And Physically

Mental and physical preparation is key to making the most of your therapy session. Mentally, be open to the experience and patient with both yourself and your horse. Therapy can be a gradual process, so setting realistic expectations is important. Physically, ensure you are in good health and capable of participating in the session's activities. Stretching and warming up before the session can help prevent injuries and improve your comfort.

Finally, practice mindfulness or relaxation techniques to help stay calm and focused during the session.

CHAPTER THREE

BUILDING A RELATIONSHIP WITH YOUR HORSE

Creating a strong bond with your horse is fundamental to successful training and a harmonious partnership.

This process involves understanding the horse's behavior, communicating effectively, and engaging in activities that build trust and mutual respect.

Here's a guide to help you simplify this process and establish a meaningful connection with your equine companion.

Techniques For Building Trust With Horses

Trust is the cornerstone of a successful relationship with your horse. Building trust begins with consistent, gentle interactions. Start by spending time near your horse without any expectations or demands. Simply being present and letting the horse come to you on its terms helps establish a sense of safety and comfort.

Use positive reinforcement techniques to encourage desired behaviors. This can involve rewarding the horse with treats, praise, or a gentle pat when they respond positively to your commands or approach. Avoid negative reinforcement or punishment, as these can damage trust and create fear.

Consistency is key. Ensure that your actions and commands are predictable and reliable. This helps the horse understand what is expected and builds confidence in your leadership.

Gradually introduce new experiences or environments in a controlled manner to help the horse become accustomed to changes without feeling overwhelmed.

Understanding Horse Behavior And Body Language

To effectively communicate with your horse, it's crucial to understand their body language and behavior. Horses are highly sensitive animals and express their feelings through their posture, ears, eyes, and overall demeanor.

Observe the horse's ears: Forward ears indicate interest or curiosity, while pinned-back ears signal irritation or discomfort.

The horse's eyes can reveal a lot about their emotional state; relaxed eyes suggest calmness, while wide eyes may indicate fear or anxiety.

Pay attention to the horse's posture and movements. A relaxed horse will exhibit a loose, swinging gait, while a tense horse may exhibit stiffness or rapid movements. By learning to read these signs, you can respond appropriately to the horse's needs and emotions.

Understanding herd dynamics can also provide insights into how your horse interacts with others. Recognizing their social behaviors and hierarchies can help you better navigate their responses and improve your overall communication.

Basic Handling And Grooming Skills

Effective handling and grooming are essential for maintaining a positive relationship with your horse. Start with basic handling skills, such as leading the horse from the ground.

Use a lead rope and walk alongside the horse, ensuring that you maintain a consistent pace and direction. Avoid pulling or jerking on the lead rope, as this can create tension.

Grooming is a great way to bond with your horse while also keeping them healthy. Use a curry comb to loosen dirt and debris from the horse's coat, followed by a stiff brush to remove the loosened material.

Be gentle and attentive to any sensitive areas, as rough handling can cause discomfort and lead to resistance.

Regular hoof care is also important. Clean the hooves daily to remove dirt and stones that can cause discomfort or injury.

Check for signs of thrush or other hoof problems, and consult a farrier for regular trims and maintenance.

Creating a positive environment for interactions is crucial for building a strong relationship with your horse.

Start by ensuring that the horse's living area is clean, safe, and comfortable. A well-maintained stall or paddock reduces stress and creates a more pleasant environment for the horse.

Establish a routine for feeding, grooming, and exercise to provide a sense of stability and predictability.

Horses thrive on routine, and consistency helps them feel secure. Avoid sudden changes to their environment or routine, as this can cause anxiety or disrupt the bond you are building.

Incorporate positive reinforcement into your interactions. Use treats, praise, or a gentle touch to reward the horse for desired behaviors.

Create a calm and soothing atmosphere during training sessions to help the horse feel relaxed and focused.

Developing A Bond Through Activities

Engaging in activities together can strengthen the bond between you and your horse. Start with simple exercises such as groundwork, which involves working with the horse from the ground to develop communication and trust. This can include exercises like leading, lunging, and desensitization to various stimuli.

Participate in activities that both you and your horse enjoy. Trail riding, for instance, can be a rewarding experience that allows you to explore new environments together.

Engage in activities that challenge and stimulate the horse mentally and physically, such as obstacle courses or agility exercises.

Regularly spending quality time with your horse, whether through training, grooming, or leisurely activities, reinforces the bond and helps build a strong, trusting relationship.

By making these experiences enjoyable and positive, you foster a deeper connection and a more harmonious partnership.

CHAPTER FOUR

EQUINE-ASSISTED THERAPY TECHNIQUES

Groundwork And Leading Exercises

Groundwork and leading exercises form the foundation of equine-assisted therapy. These activities focus on building trust, communication, and coordination between the horse and the therapist. To start, it's crucial to establish a safe and comfortable environment for both the horse and the participant. Begin with simple leading exercises where the participant learns how to guide the horse using a lead rope. This helps in developing leadership skills and enhances the participant's confidence.

Exercises like "following the leader" involve the participant leading the horse through a series of obstacles or patterns.

These tasks encourage focus, coordination, and responsiveness. The therapist should guide the participant in maintaining appropriate body posture and using clear, consistent cues. As the participant becomes more proficient, they can progress to more complex groundwork activities such as lateral movements and walking in specific patterns.

Another essential aspect of groundwork is teaching the participant to groom and handle the horse. This involves brushing, cleaning hooves, and performing basic health checks. These activities not only foster a bond between the participant and the horse but also develop fine motor skills and attention to detail.

Riding And Mounted Activities

Riding and mounted activities offer significant therapeutic benefits by combining physical exercise with emotional and cognitive challenges. Starting with basic mounting techniques, participants learn how to safely get on and off the horse. This process should be broken down into manageable steps, ensuring that the participant feels secure and comfortable.

Once mounted, participants engage in various riding exercises that enhance their balance, coordination, and strength. Simple activities like walking in circles or riding over poles can be introduced to improve motor skills and spatial awareness. The therapist should focus on ensuring that the participant maintains proper posture and utilizes their core muscles effectively.

Mounted activities can also include more advanced maneuvers such as trotting or cantering, depending on the participant's skill level and comfort.

Riding exercises are tailored to individual needs and goals, with adjustments made based on the participant's progress and feedback. Incorporating patterns or specific routes can help improve cognitive functions such as memory and concentration.

Sensory And Balance Exercises

Sensory and balance exercises are designed to enhance the participant's sensory integration and proprioceptive awareness. These exercises involve interacting with the horse in ways that stimulate different senses and challenge balance.

For sensory exercises, participants might engage in activities such as brushing the horse with different textured brushes or walking alongside the horse while blindfolded.

 These activities help in improving tactile sensitivity and spatial awareness. The therapist should guide how to safely and effectively engage with these sensory experiences.

Balance exercises often include activities like riding with one hand off the reins or performing gentle exercises while mounted, such as reaching for objects or performing simple stretches.

These exercises are aimed at improving the participant's core strength and overall stability. The therapist needs to monitor the participant's balance and adjust the difficulty of the exercises as needed.

Therapeutic Games And Challenges

Therapeutic games and challenges add an element of fun and motivation to the therapy sessions. These activities are designed to reinforce therapeutic goals while engaging the participant in enjoyable and interactive tasks.

Examples of therapeutic games include obstacle courses, where participants guide the horse through various challenges, or "Simon Says" with horse-related commands. These games promote problem-solving skills, coordination, and responsiveness. The therapist should create a variety of games that align with the participant's therapeutic goals and skill level.

Challenges can be tailored to address specific areas of development, such as improving fine motor skills or cognitive functions. For instance, participants might work on tasks that require them to retrieve objects from the ground while riding or perform specific patterns with the horse. These challenges encourage engagement and perseverance while reinforcing therapeutic objectives.

Customizing Techniques For Individual Needs

Customizing equine-assisted therapy techniques to individual needs is crucial for maximizing the effectiveness of the therapy. Each participant has unique goals, abilities, and challenges, and the treatment should be tailored accordingly.

Start by conducting a thorough assessment of the participant's needs and goals. This involves understanding their physical abilities, emotional state, and any specific therapeutic objectives. Based on this assessment, the therapist can design a personalized therapy plan that includes appropriate groundwork, riding activities, sensory exercises, and therapeutic games.

Regularly review and adjust the therapy plan based on the participant's progress and feedback. This might involve modifying exercises to increase their complexity or introducing new activities to keep the participant engaged.

The therapist should maintain open communication with the participant and any other involved caregivers to ensure that the therapy remains aligned with the participant's evolving needs and goals.

CHAPTER FIVE

ADDRESSING EMOTIONAL AND PSYCHOLOGICAL ISSUES

Using Horses To Manage Anxiety And Depression

Horses have an extraordinary ability to sense and respond to human emotions, making them exceptional partners in managing anxiety and depression.

Interacting with horses can create a calming environment that helps alleviate symptoms of these mental health challenges.

When working with horses, individuals often experience a reduction in stress levels due to the animal's serene presence and non-judgmental nature.

Grooming a horse, for instance, provides a repetitive, soothing activity that can distract from anxious thoughts and provide a sense of calm.

Additionally, the physical activity involved in caring for a horse, such as walking or riding, can release endorphins and improve mood.

The process involves building a relationship with the horse, which can lead to increased feelings of safety and trust.

This bond often helps individuals open up about their feelings and experiences, making it easier to address underlying issues.

Structured equine therapy sessions, guided by trained professionals, can incorporate specific techniques designed to address anxiety and depression, such as mindfulness exercises, goal-setting, and reflective practices.

Therapeutic Techniques For Trauma Recovery

Equine therapy is particularly effective for trauma recovery due to its ability to provide a safe space for individuals to process and heal from past experiences.

Horses can help individuals reconnect with their emotions and gain insight into their trauma through various therapeutic techniques.

One common approach is to use horses in ground activities that do not require riding. These activities focus on building trust and communication between the individual and the horse.

For example, leading a horse through obstacle courses or engaging in groundwork exercises can parallel the individual's journey through emotional obstacles.

Therapists often use the horse's reactions to help individuals understand and confront their trauma.

For example, if a horse reacts nervously to a certain behavior or command, it can help the individual recognize their triggers and responses.

Through this interaction, individuals can learn to manage their reactions and work through their trauma in a supportive environment.

Another technique involves using horse behavior as a mirror for personal behavior. By observing and interacting with the horse, individuals can gain insights into their emotional states and patterns, facilitating deeper self-awareness and healing.

Building Self-Esteem And Confidence Through Interaction

Interacting with horses can be a powerful tool for building self-esteem and confidence. The process of working with a horse requires and fosters skills such as leadership, responsibility, and patience, all of which contribute to a person's self-worth.

Tasks such as grooming, feeding, and training a horse provide opportunities for individuals to set and achieve goals. Completing these tasks can boost self-confidence and foster a sense of accomplishment. For example, teaching a horse a new trick or mastering a specific riding technique can be a significant confidence builder.

Additionally, the unconditional acceptance of a horse helps individuals feel valued and respected, which can enhance self-esteem.

Horses do not judge or criticize; they respond to the individual's actions and emotions, providing positive reinforcement and encouragement.

Therapeutic activities often include setting personal goals related to horse care or riding, which helps individuals experience tangible progress and success. These achievements can translate into increased self-confidence and a more positive self-image.

Equine-Assisted Techniques For Social Skills Development

Equine-assisted therapy can play a crucial role in developing social skills by providing a dynamic and interactive environment. Working with horses requires effective communication and cooperation, which can translate into improved social skills in other areas of life.

Activities such as leading a horse, coordinating movements, and following instructions help individuals practice and enhance their communication abilities. For example, learning how to give clear commands to a horse or working together with others in a group setting can improve verbal and non-verbal communication skills.

Horses also help individuals practice empathy and understanding. Interacting with a horse requires recognizing and responding to the animal's needs and emotions, which can enhance an individual's ability to connect with others on a deeper level. This empathetic connection fosters better relationships and social interactions outside of the equine setting.

Group therapy sessions with horses can also provide opportunities for individuals to work on teamwork and collaboration. Activities that involve group problem-solving or cooperative exercises with horses can strengthen social bonds and improve interpersonal skills.

Tracking Emotional Progress And Success

Monitoring emotional progress and success in equine therapy involves tracking changes in behavior, mood, and overall well-being. This can be done through various methods, including self-reports, therapist observations, and structured assessments.

Keeping a journal of interactions and feelings during therapy sessions can help individuals and therapists identify patterns and progress. Regularly recording experiences and emotions can provide valuable insights into how equine therapy is impacting emotional health.

Therapists often use specific assessment tools to measure changes in anxiety, depression, and overall emotional well-being. These tools can include standardized questionnaires, behavioral observations, and goal-setting evaluations. By comparing these assessments over time, individuals and therapists can gauge the effectiveness of the therapy and make adjustments as needed.

Celebrating milestones and achievements in therapy is also important for tracking success. Recognizing and acknowledging progress, no matter how small, can motivate individuals and reinforce the positive impact of equine-assisted therapy on their emotional and psychological well-being.

CHAPTER SIX

PHYSICAL BENEFITS OF EQUINE-ASSISTED THERAPY

Equine-assisted therapy (EAT) offers a variety of physical benefits, significantly impacting participants' overall well-being. Here's a detailed look at how interacting with horses can lead to physical improvements:

Improving Balance And Coordination

One of the key physical benefits of EAT is the enhancement of balance and coordination. When riding or interacting with horses, individuals engage their core muscles and maintain balance while adjusting to the horse's movements. This dynamic activity requires continuous fine-tuning of motor responses, which improves overall body awareness. The rhythmic motion of the horse mimics natural walking patterns, helping riders develop better balance and coordination as they learn to stabilize themselves on an unpredictable surface. This practice is particularly beneficial for those with neurological conditions or balance impairments.

Enhancing Motor Skills And Physical Strength

Equine-assisted therapy can significantly enhance motor skills and physical strength. Riding a horse involves a range of motor tasks, from controlling the reins to maneuvering the horse and maintaining posture. These activities require and build both gross and fine motor skills. For instance, steering a horse requires precise hand movements and coordination between the rider's legs and hands. Additionally, the physical effort of maintaining posture and engaging core muscles during a ride strengthens the lower back, abdomen, and legs. This increased physical strength supports better overall fitness and muscular endurance.

Pain Management And Rehabilitation Support

EAT is also beneficial for pain management and rehabilitation support. The gentle, rhythmic motion of the horse can have therapeutic effects, helping to alleviate pain and stiffness in muscles and joints.

The consistent movement and warmth of the horse's body can act as a form of passive exercise, reducing muscle tension and promoting relaxation. For those undergoing rehabilitation, EAT offers a motivating and enjoyable way to engage in physical activity, which can accelerate recovery and enhance overall mobility. The supportive and non-judgmental environment provided by horses can also contribute to reduced stress and pain levels.

Techniques For Developing Physical Endurance

Developing physical endurance through EAT involves a variety of techniques. Regular riding sessions require sustained physical effort, which helps build cardiovascular endurance and muscular stamina.

Riders can engage in specific exercises such as trotting or cantering to increase heart rate and endurance levels. Structured therapy sessions often include a combination of riding and ground exercises, such as grooming and leading the horse, to enhance overall physical conditioning.

These activities not only improve endurance but also boost overall fitness levels by integrating strength, flexibility, and cardiovascular health.

Assessing Physical Progress And Health Benefits

Assessing physical progress in EAT involves monitoring various health indicators and functional improvements. Progress can be evaluated through regular physical assessments, such as measuring balance, coordination, strength, and endurance before and after therapy sessions. Observations of increased stability, improved muscle tone, and enhanced motor skills can indicate positive changes. Additionally, subjective measures such as reduced pain levels and increased participation in daily activities reflect the therapeutic benefits of EAT. Regular feedback from therapists and participants helps to track improvements and adjust therapy plans to maximize health benefits.

CHAPTER SEVEN

COMMON CHALLENGES AND SOLUTIONS

Overcoming Fear And Anxiety Around Horses

One of the primary hurdles when starting equine therapy is overcoming fear and anxiety, whether it's from the client or the horse.

 For clients, this fear often stems from past experiences or misconceptions about horses. To address this, begin with gradual exposure in a controlled environment.

Start by observing the horses from a safe distance, allowing clients to get accustomed to their presence without direct interaction.

Introduce clients to the horses slowly, using positive reinforcement techniques to build trust.

Encourage them to participate in non-threatening tasks such as grooming or feeding the horse, which helps create a positive association with the animals. Additionally, providing education about horse behavior and safety can alleviate fears.

Techniques such as deep breathing and mindfulness exercises can also help manage anxiety during sessions.

For horses, fear and anxiety might manifest as nervous behavior or aggression. Understanding and addressing the root cause of these behaviors is crucial.

A professional horse trainer or behaviorist can work with the horse to build its confidence and reduce fear through consistent, positive reinforcement training. Establishing a calm, predictable routine for the horse also helps in reducing anxiety.

Addressing Behavioral Issues In Horses

Behavioral issues in horses can range from minor annoyances to significant problems that impact the effectiveness of therapy sessions. Common issues include biting, kicking, or refusal to cooperate.

Identifying the cause of these behaviors is the first step toward resolution. This might involve observing the horse's interactions with its environment, other horses, and humans to pinpoint triggers.

Training and desensitization are key strategies for managing behavioral problems. Positive reinforcement, such as rewards for calm behavior, can be effective in encouraging desirable actions. Consistency in handling and clear communication with the horse also plays a crucial role in modifying behavior. Regularly scheduled training sessions with a qualified instructor can further support the horse in developing better habits.

In some cases, behavioral issues may stem from physical discomfort or health problems. Ensuring the horse is regularly checked by a veterinarian can rule out medical causes and ensure the horse's well-being.

Managing Session Disruptions And Setbacks

Disruptions and setbacks can occur in any therapeutic setting and can be challenging to manage.

Common disruptions might include unexpected behavior from the horse, client difficulties, or external factors such as weather changes.

Planning and flexibility are essential in dealing with these issues.

Have a contingency plan in place for dealing with disruptions. This might involve having alternate activities or exercises that can be substituted if the planned session cannot proceed as expected. Keeping communication open with clients and discussing any issues that arise can help in managing expectations and reducing frustration.

If a setback occurs, such as a regression in progress, assess the situation calmly and make necessary adjustments.

This might involve altering the therapy plan or taking a step back to address underlying issues.

Continuous evaluation and adaptation of the therapy process help in maintaining progress and overcoming challenges.

Adapting Therapy Techniques For Special Needs

Special needs clients may require modifications to standard therapy techniques to ensure the sessions are effective and comfortable. These adaptations might include adjusting the intensity of the exercises, using specialized equipment, or providing additional support.

For clients with physical disabilities, consider modifications that accommodate their needs, such as providing support harnesses or using adaptive equipment to facilitate their interaction with the horse. Communication is crucial; ensure that you understand the specific needs and preferences of the client to tailor the therapy accordingly.

In the case of cognitive or emotional special needs, the focus should be on creating a supportive and understanding environment. Use clear, simple instructions, and be patient. Adapt the pace of the sessions to match the client's comfort level and ensure that they feel secure and supported throughout the process.

Troubleshooting Common Issues In Therapy

During equine therapy, various common issues may arise, such as difficulty in establishing rapport with the horse, challenges in maintaining the client's engagement, or issues with achieving therapy goals. Identifying and addressing these issues promptly is key to a successful therapeutic experience.

If establishing rapport with the horse is difficult, consider revisiting basic training exercises to build a stronger bond. Increasing the amount of positive interaction and using treats or praise can help in improving the horse's response.

For client engagement, it's important to keep sessions varied and interesting. Incorporate different activities and regularly check in with clients to understand their interests and preferences. Adjusting the therapy goals to be more realistic and achievable can also help in maintaining motivation and progress.

Regular feedback sessions with clients and ongoing assessments of the therapy process are crucial for identifying and resolving issues. By maintaining a flexible approach and being open to adjustments, you can effectively manage common challenges and ensure the success of equine therapy.

CHAPTER EIGHT

INTEGRATING EQUINE THERAPY INTO YOUR LIFE

Creating A Routine With Regular Therapy Sessions

Integrating equine therapy into your life starts with establishing a consistent routine. Begin by scheduling regular therapy sessions that fit into your weekly or bi-weekly calendar. Consistency is key to maximizing the benefits of equine therapy, as frequent interaction with horses fosters deeper emotional connections and reinforces therapeutic progress.

Consider setting specific days and times for your sessions to create a predictable schedule. This routine helps your mind and body adjust to the therapy, making each session more effective. Work closely with your therapist to determine the best frequency for your needs, and remember that flexibility is essential. Life can be unpredictable, so having a flexible routine ensures you can adjust without losing momentum.

Combining Therapy With Other Treatments

Equine therapy can be an excellent complement to other forms of treatment, such as physical therapy, psychotherapy, or medication. To make the most of this integrative approach, collaborate with your healthcare providers to develop a comprehensive treatment plan. This plan should align your equine therapy goals with those of your other treatments, ensuring that all aspects of your care are working synergistically.

For example, if you are undergoing physical therapy for a specific condition, discuss how equine therapy can complement these exercises. Horses can help improve balance, coordination, and strength, which might enhance your progress in physical therapy. Similarly, if you are working through emotional challenges with a therapist, equine therapy can offer additional support and emotional release.

Setting Long-Term Goals And Tracking Progress

Setting clear, long-term goals for your equine therapy is crucial for measuring progress and maintaining motivation. Start by identifying what you hope to achieve through therapy. These goals might include improving emotional well-being, enhancing physical abilities, or developing new skills with horses.

Once you have established your goals, work with your therapist to create a plan for reaching them. Regularly review and adjust this plan based on your progress. Tracking your achievements, no matter how small, helps you stay focused and motivated. Keep a journal or use an app to document your experiences, track changes in your condition, and celebrate milestones.

Involving Family and Support Systems

Involving your family and support systems in your equine therapy journey can enhance its effectiveness. Share your goals and progress with those close to you, so they understand your therapy's importance and can offer encouragement. Family members can also participate in sessions or activities, which can strengthen bonds and foster a supportive environment.

Additionally, educate your family and friends about the benefits of equine therapy. Understanding the process and its impact can help them provide better support and be more involved in your journey. Encourage open communication about your experiences and any adjustments needed in your therapy routine.

Maintaining The Benefits Outside Of Sessions

To maintain the benefits of equine therapy outside of your sessions, integrate the lessons learned into your daily life.

Apply the coping strategies, physical exercises, and emotional insights gained during therapy to your routine.

For instance, if you've learned relaxation techniques while working with horses, practice them during stressful moments at home or work.

Incorporate activities that reinforce the skills developed during therapy, such as engaging in physical exercise or participating in social events that support your emotional well-being. Keeping a positive mindset and staying active in your therapy principles can help sustain the progress you've made and continue benefiting from equine therapy.

CHAPTER NINE

COMMON CONCERNS AND DETAILED FAQS

What If I've Never Been Around Horses Before?

It's completely normal to feel apprehensive if you've never been around horses before. Many people who start equine-assisted therapy have little to no experience with horses. Your first step will typically involve getting comfortable with the horse and the environment. The therapy sessions are designed to be welcoming and educational, ensuring you feel at ease.

You will begin by learning basic horse handling skills, which include grooming, leading, and understanding horse behavior. This foundational knowledge helps build trust between you and the horse. Your therapist will guide you through every step, offering clear instructions and support. With patience and time, most people find that they quickly overcome their initial apprehension and develop a positive bond with the horse.

How Do I Know If Equine Therapy Is Right For Me?

Determining if equine therapy is right for you involves considering your personal goals and needs. Equine therapy is beneficial for various issues, including emotional challenges, physical rehabilitation, and developmental disorders. If you're seeking a unique approach to address these concerns or are looking for alternative therapies, equine therapy might be a good fit.

Discuss your goals and any specific needs with your therapist during an initial consultation. They will assess your situation and help you understand how equine therapy can be integrated into your overall treatment plan.

This initial evaluation is crucial in tailoring the therapy to ensure it aligns with your objectives and maximizes the potential benefits.

What Are The Costs Associated With Equine-Assisted Therapy?

The costs of equine-assisted therapy can vary depending on several factors, including the therapist's qualifications, the duration and frequency of sessions, and the location of the therapy center. Typically, prices can range from $75 to $150 per session, but this can vary widely.

Insurance coverage for equine therapy may also differ based on your provider and plan. Some insurance plans cover a portion of the costs, especially if the therapy is prescribed by a healthcare professional. It's advisable to contact your insurance company to understand your coverage and any out-of-pocket expenses you might incur.

How Do I Choose The Right Therapist For My Needs?

Selecting the right therapist is essential for a successful equine-assisted therapy experience. Start by researching therapists who specialize in equine therapy and have the necessary credentials and experience. Look for professionals who are certified in equine therapy and have a strong background in working with the specific issues you want to address.

It's beneficial to schedule a consultation to discuss your needs and evaluate the therapist's approach. During this meeting, ask about their experience, therapy methods, and the horses they work with. The right therapist will be someone who listens to your concerns, answers your questions thoroughly, and makes you feel comfortable and confident in your care.

What Are The Risks And How Are They Managed?

Like any therapeutic activity involving animals, equine-assisted therapy carries some inherent risks. These might include the potential for falls, bites, or kicks, as well as allergic reactions or anxiety related to interacting with large animals. However, these risks are generally minimal and manageable with proper precautions.

Therapists are trained to handle horses safely and to ensure that clients are protected during sessions. They will guide how to interact with the horse safely and will always supervise the sessions closely. Additionally, horses used in therapy are carefully selected for their temperament and suitability for therapeutic work. By adhering to safety protocols and working with experienced professionals, the risks are effectively minimized, allowing you to focus on the therapeutic benefits.